Reloaded: Natural Hair Loss Secrets for Safe, Effective Hair Growth

Reloaded: Natural Hair Loss Secrets for Safe, Effective Hair Growth

David Rodgers, M.S. Nutrition

Published by Clear Stone Press, 2011

Copyright © 2011 David Rodgers

Published by Clear Stone Press

No part of this publication may be reproduced, stored in a
retrieval system, or transmitted in any form or by any means,
electronic, mechanical, photocopying, recording, scanning, or
otherwise, except with permission of the publisher, or except as
permitted under Section 107 or 108 of the 1976 United States
Copyright Act.

All rights reserved.

ISBN: 061556383X
ISBN-13: 978-0615563831

DEDICATION

To my wife, Beth, my parents, and my family, who have been very supportive of my quest to find and report the truth about natural health.

ACKNOWLEDGMENTS

A thank you goes out to those health professionals who have an open mind and are willing to speak the truth about the incredible benefits of natural health therapies, even when they are not popular or widely accepted yet. Such professionals are Dr. Joesph Mercola, Dr. Mehmet Oz, Dr. Al Sears, Dr. James Balch, Dr. Mark Stengler, Jonny Bowden, M.S., Dr. Sandra Cabot, and many others.

TABLE OF CONTENTS

Reloaded: Natural Hair Loss Secrets for Safe, Effective Hair Growth

INTRODUCTION

As a reader, I am always happier when authors get to the meat of the topic right away. Therefore, this introduction will be very brief. My name is David Rodgers, I have a Master's of Science in human nutrition from the University of Bridgeport, and I spend my free time researching scientifically proven natural remedies for many different conditions. In the case of hair loss, the current mainstream dogma is that nothing re-grows hair except for Rogaine and Propecia. I'm here to tell you that this is scientifically false.

Many of the items in this book have been scientifically proven and verified to not only stop hair loss, but also to re-grow it. Others are based on scientifically proven ideas, but the actual linkage to hair loss is not yet verified. Lastly, some of the items are only included due to individual testing and testimonials, which I will admit is unscientific. However, I believe that when finally tested scientifically, the majority of these unproven methods will also be proven and verified. Until that time, people need a variety of options for naturally re-growing hair, and as these currently unproven methods have certainly proven to not be harmful in the least, I thought it would be a mistake to leave them out.

Through extensive research, I have concluded that there are four main reasons for hair loss, and sometimes two or more of these reasons overlap, or in some cases one is the cause of another. The four are: nutrient deficiencies, thyroid hormone imbalance, prostate hormone imbalance, and calcification. As almost all of the methods listed in this book are entirely safe and inexpensive, it would be worth your while to give most of them a try. Many people would be surprised to find that for most of the therapies, it is evident whether they will work or not within a couple weeks (not months).

In addition to the four sections highlighting the four main causes of hair loss, I have also included a fifth section which highlights various other proven and unproven hair growth methods. That section also touches on help for autoimmune-related hair loss (which could be considered a fifth cause) that often comes out in patches and is called alopecia arreata.

Near the conclusion of the book, I have included a table which rates every single one of the therapies mentioned based on five criteria: scientific evidence, prevalence of web testimonials, the author's (my own) experience with the product, the expense of the therapy, and other (non-hair) positive health effects. This table should help you select the best therapies based on your areas of concern. Also included in the table is the method of the therapy, which includes instructions on what to buy, dosages, recommended brand names, and how to take the therapy.

Please note that this book is intended to help both men and women combat hair loss. However, there are a few recommendations that are for men only. These can all be found in chapter three. All other recommendations are for both sexes (all are applicable to men and none are only for women).

Also, please note that each recommendation is aimed at a specific cause of hair loss. Some recommendations will work for some but not for others because they might, for example, be aimed at correcting a situation that was not imbalanced in the first place.

CAUTION

Although the recommendations in this book are largely dietary and/or over-the-counter in nature, it is prudent to first check with your doctor, especially if you are concurrently taking drugs and wish to add dietary supplements. This should help guard against possible drug-nutrient interactions. You may start dosages small to assess and avoid possible (though mild and unlikely) side effects. Discontinue usage if side effects continue.

SPECIAL OFFER

I am looking for before and after pictures showing noticeable hair growth using only methods described in this book. These can be taken in anonymous fashion from the top of the head (like those on this book's cover). However, it is also nice to see a real face if you aren't shy. For those who send pictures, I am offering $15 off the purchase of a nutrition consultation by phone/video conference (transferable to friends or family). Send digital photos to nutrientbalance@gmail.com - thanks!

1. NUTRIENT DEFICIENCY

Protein / Hemp Protein

Hair is made out of several minerals, compounds, and nutrients, but the primary component is a protein called keratin. Those suffering from dietary protein deficiency might find their hair not as thick or full as they remember. The mainstream medical opinion on protein is that "nearly all" Americans get enough. I would agree that a majority of Americans do consume adequate protein, but the numbers are not as high as "nearly all." Those deficient in protein are more likely to be vegetarian or vegan, or those trying to be as healthy as possible (however this is certainly not always the case). Also, as we will see below, it is important to not only consume enough protein, but also to absorb enough, which doesn't always happen in the elderly or those with compromised gastrointestinal tract health.

A study from the American Journal of Clinical Nutrition was done on 95 medicare-aged patients, and it was found that deficient protein intake is correlated with inadequate anagen hair protein, which is the protein found at the root/bulb of the hair, or the most important part for growth. Not only was this the case, but it was also found that inadequate protein intake showed up in laboratory results as a deficit in hair protein before a deficit showed in other protein markers such as albumin (a protein commonly measured in the blood). This means that the body is prioritizing protein for areas that it deems as most vitally important. While the look of your hair may be vitally important to your psychological needs, the body sees the hair as secondary to your internal health needs; therefore, your hair is the first item to show damage. [1]

So, the question at this point becomes, "how can I make sure that I am getting enough protein?" The answer comes from some equations that you can do on a simple calculator. For inactive individuals, one recommended protein intake guideline that I agree with is 1.2 grams per kilogram of body weight per day. [2] In individuals with chronic inflammation or disease, the intake should be 1.5 grams per kilogram per day. Active individuals, and especially those who train with weights or use muscles to the point of soreness on a regular basis, will need more protein, perhaps in the range of 1.5-1.8 grams per kilogram per day.

To find your specific optimal amount, take your weight in pounds and divide by 2.2 to get your weight in kilograms. Then take that kilogram weight and multiply by your optimal amount per day, which should be 1.2, 1.5, or 1.8. Your final answer is the amount in grams of protein you should be consuming in a day. Be sure to count based on nutrition facts labels. If the labels aren't available, you can go by these simplified rules: 4 ounces of chicken, beef, turkey, or fish, which is sized at a little bigger than a deck of cards has around 20-24 grams of protein. A handful of nuts or seeds, or a half-cup of cooked lentils, has around 8 grams of protein.

For an easy way to reach the optimal protein amount, I recommend hemp protein powder, as it is one of the only protein powders that is raw, contains all of the enzymes necessary to digest, and also contains a significant amount of beneficial fiber and essential fatty acids.

Hemp protein powder does not have the best taste in the world, but it is not terrible, and it can be stirred into water without any additional flavorings. It can also be added to smoothies or shakes, but be aware that it will make these drinks much thicker and probably not quite as tasty.

Regarding my own experience with hair loss, adding protein in general did not appear to have a huge effect. However, adding hemp protein specifically does seem to add to thickness and strength. No research currently backs up hemp specifically. However, it is interesting to note that hemp is also used to make very strong ropes and other hair-like non-food products. There are testimonials for both internal and topically-applied hemp protein and hemp oil regarding hair loss and hair strength throughout the web. Therefore, even if you are not protein deficient, it would be a good idea to try a scoopful or more of hemp protein (which also contains hemp oil and beneficial minerals and fiber as well) per day.

I also mentioned the idea of absorption, and this is important, because protein can be consumed all day long, but if it isn't absorbed and assimilated into the body, and therefore into the hair, one can still be in a state of protein deficiency. There are two main factors to consider when assessing protein absorption: insulin levels and gastrointestinal health.

When one eats any type of sugar or carbohydrate (except for fiber), insulin is secreted in the bloodstream. Insulin is an anabolic hormone, because it causes a state of growth in the body. Insulin takes raw materials from your food and deposits them in cells around the body. While of course, insulin deposits sugar and carbohydrates, it also delivers fat and protein to cells.

It is important to note that if the body has had few or no carbs for a significant portion of time, there will be no "shuttle service" for protein to find its way into the muscles, and everywhere else in the body, including the hair. Therefore, in order to absorb protein, be sure to also consume a moderate amount of carbs at the same time or shortly before.

The second issue regarding protein absorption is gastrointestinal health. As this is not a book on gastrointestinal function, I won't go into much detail here. What I will make note of is that digestive enzymes are often a very significant help, even for people who have a totally healthy GI tract. For those who don't have healthy GI function, digestive enzymes can be even more crucial.

You may recall from science class that enzymes are molecules that help to catalyze, or spur on, a chemical reaction. When the body has a difficult time digesting protein, it often means that these enzymes are not present in sufficient quantities to catalyze the reactions of digestion. Therefore, food that is not broken down well enough is passed from the stomach into the small and then large intestines, and it eventually leaves the body. The result is a feeling of weakness, muscularly and otherwise, a decline in immune function, and a lack of resources for other parts of the body, but most notably, the hair.

In order to restore digestive enzymes, simply find a supplement from a health food store that contains protease enzymes. A good amount of protease would be 20,000 USP (United States Pharmacopeia) units per pill. Digestive enzymes often include a variety of other ingredients that help to break down food. Amylase is the enzyme that breaks down carbohydrates and lipase is the enzyme that breaks down fatty acids. Bromelain is one form of a protease enzyme that comes from pineapple; similarly, papain is a protease enzyme from papaya.

Follow the serving size listed on the bottle of digestive enzymes; however, usually it is best to take them just before or at the beginning of a meal. This gets the stomach and intestines fully prepared to digest the protein just before it receives it.

Essential Fatty Acids and Other Beneficial Fats

Many Americans are lacking in enough essential fatty acids, and I would estimate that the majority of Americans are lacking in quality versions of these fatty acids. Rather than quality oils, they consume over-processed, overheated, and genetically modified versions found in most grocery stores and restaurants.

For simplicity's sake, there are five types of fatty acids: omega 3, omega 6, omega 9, saturated, and trans/hydrogenated fatty acids. Of those, four are natural to the body and beneficial to health when consumed in the correct quantities. Trans fats, or hydrogenated oils, on the other hand, are chemically altered slow poisons, which means that they don't kill you right away, but with moderate to high consumption over time, your cells become poisoned by artificial materials, and heart disease and various other chronic diseases are inevitable.

To avoid trans fats, simply don't eat anything deep fried, anything that lists any amount of trans fats on a nutrition label, or any item that lists "hydrogenated" anything, "partially," "fully," or otherwise, in the ingredients. Yes, this involves giving up French fries in favor of baked potatoes, and giving up chicken nuggets and getting baked chicken instead. Your whole body and hair will thank you and you will likely live longer as a result.

Of those five types of fats listed above, two are called essential fatty acids: omega 3 and omega 6. "Essential" means that it is crucial that you consume them in your diet, because the body can't produce them from other fats or carbs. You likely know that omega 3 comes from fish, fish oil, flax seeds, walnuts, etc. Omega 6 fats in the American diet largely come from unhealthy sources such as corn oil, canola oil, cottonseed oil, and soybean oil. All four of these oils are highly processed and largely come from genetically-modified sources, unless they were purchased at a health food store and the label says otherwise ("cold-pressed" or "non-GMO" are healthy labels, as is "organic").

Instead, you should be getting your omega 6 oils from healthy, non-processed sources. The best sources are raw walnuts (which also contain omega 3), raw sunflower seeds, cold-pressed sunflower oil, or cold-pressed sesame oil. In order to achieve your optimal amount per day, you should have 1-2 handfuls of the nuts or seeds, or 1-2 tablespoons of the oils.

I must mention that many sources, including both conventional and natural-minded health experts, often argue that omega 6 fatty acids are negative for health, as they lead to a state of inflammation. It is argued that a lower omega 6 to omega 3 ratio is healthier. I do agree that most people would be healthier with a larger amount of omega 3, but I disagree with the universal denouncing of omega 6 fats.

I counter the teachings of these experts by explaining that inflammatory effects completely depend on the source of the oil. Those oils that I listed two paragraphs above are generally said to be healthy despite the fact that they largely contain omega 6 oils. More information on omega 6 benefits can be found in my free online report, "Diet Soda Makes You Fatter Than Regular and 10 More Shocking Health Truths." You can download it at nutrientbalance.com/dietsodareport.

If you cook with these oils, or any oils, be sure to stay below the smokepoint of the oils. The smokepoint is the temperature at which the oils begin to smoke, and can turn into trans fats. To find smokepoints, simply Google the oil you are using along with the term smokepoint, and you'll see it. For example, you would use the search term "sunflower oil smokepoint" to find the highest temperature you should ever use to cook sunflower oil. There are often different smokepoints listed on different sites. Not all sites are reputable, so choose those that appear more reputable, or if you are unsure, then use the lowest listed smokepoint to be safe. It is better to cook for longer periods at a lower, safer temperature than to cook for shorter periods at a high temperature. Plus, this usually tastes better because you aren't burning portions of your food. Burnt food in general, but especially burnt meat, can be carcinogenic, so cut off these portions if necessary.

In regards to omega 3, the optimal type you should be consuming is fish oil, which contains EPA and DHA, the main forms of omega 3 that are active in the body. Choose a brand that is molecularly distilled (this will be indicated on the bottle) because this process is effective in removing mercury and other toxins. Find out the total amount of EPA and DHA per pill and take enough pills to equal 1200 to 2000mg per day. Some brands have pills that contain larger amounts of EPA and DHA, such as Jarrow EPA-DHA Balance, or Natural Factors RxOmega 3 Factors. If you buy either of these two products, you would only need two or three pills per day, as opposed to

4-6 or even more from many other types of fish oil products.

There is no direct evidence at this time that essential fatty acids re-grow hair (future studies will likely prove that it is true). However I have included them for a couple reasons. The first is that they have been proven to partially block testosterone from being converted to dihydro-testosterone or DHT [3] [4] [5] (I will explain this later). The second is that reputable organizations often correlate essentially fatty acid deficiency with dry hair, or poor hair growth. [6]

Regarding testosterone and the conversion to DHT, this has been shown to be one of the factors behind prostate enlargement and hair loss for men. We will go much more into detail on this in the section on prostate hormones. However, for now I will simply say that eating the right amount of fats, especially omega 3 and omega 6, but also omega 9 and certain saturated fats, is the easiest and most natural way to lower or normalize the conversion of testosterone to DHT, which will directly help keep hair on one's head and help to restore health to the prostate gland.

Although women generally do not have the same issue regarding DHT (they only have a very small amount), I do still make all of the same recommendations regarding essential fatty acids and other dietary corrections outlined in this chapter. In fact, everyone (even those not affected by hair loss), would be healthier if they were to follow these recommendations because dietary deficiencies affect not only hair, but also every cell in the body. However, regarding the DHT issue, there are three main recommendations in chapter three that women can ignore, as they are more intently focused on prostate health correction which, in their case, is not necessary.

Gamma Linolenic Acid

There are many types of omega 3 and omega 6 fatty acids, but the "mother" fatty acid for omega 3 is the plant-based alpha linolenic acid or ALA, (found in flax seeds, chia seeds, walnuts, etc.), and for omega 6 it is linoleic acid or LA, (found in many nuts and seeds including sesame, sunflower, and pumpkin seeds, pecans, etc). The "mother" fatty acid means that all other omega

3 or 6 fatty acids begin there and are converted accordingly. Most animal forms of omega 3 have already been converted from ALA into the more active forms of EPA and DHA (two of the most important fatty acids you find in fish oil and grass-fed, but not conventional beef).

When you consume the plant based ALA, a small amount of it is converted into EPA and DHA in your body, however many experts recommend that you consume EPA and DHA directly so that you don't have to rely on a conversion mechanism to get the nutrients you need. These experts argue that many people don't have the proper gastrointestinal health to make the ALA to DHA/EPA conversion, and others don't consume enough ALA to have the raw materials for the conversion to take place.

Just as the omega 3 plant-based "mother" ALA makes the conversion into EPA and DHA, the omega six "mother," linolenic acid gets converted into gamma linolenic acid (GLA) and then arachidonic acid (AA) in the body. Also similarly, many experts believe that the conversion process is not always working in tip-top shape, in which case, supplementing with GLA may be a wise option. (Dietary arachidonic acid, or AA, is more prevalent in the diet and not needed as a supplement).

GLA comes in the form of borage oil, evening primrose oil, or black currant seed oil supplements, because these are among the few foods that have a significant amount of GLA. Hemp powder and spirulina have a smaller amount. If you are interested in trying GLA, I recommend getting a brand that has a GLA content of 240mg per pill (Jarrow and Source Naturals are good choices). Many companies have pills with the GLA content in the range of 40-60mg, which is not enough to make a difference. Even 240mg is a small amount when you consider that if you consume a handful of walnuts, you are getting 11,000mg of linoleic acid (LA).

However, men should not take more than one 240mg pill per day, because according to various sources - although none fully backed up by a peer-reviewed study - evening primrose oil may have estrogenic activity. [7] I was unable to find this same link when searching for borage oil or black currant seed oil, however in general, evening primrose, black currant, and borage oil all have similar testimonials in regards to helping PMS symptoms, breast tenderness, and more. Therefore, for males at least, it is probably a good idea to exercise caution and not take a large dose of GLA. Women should limit to two 240mg pills per day.

I recommend that it is worth trying GLA for the same reasons as general omega 3 and 6. First, it is because GLA can also help normalize the conversion of testosterone into DHT. In fact, GLA is more potent than any of the other fatty acids in this regard. [3] Second, it is because GLA is often quoted for its beneficial effects on hair health (although this has not been officially researched). There are also a significant amount of positive web testimonials regarding the usage of GLA for hair health.

Omega 9 and Saturated Fats

I should mention that after omega 3 and omega 6 fatty acids have been consumed in sufficient quantities, the best oils to consume for general health are cold pressed olive oil or raw almonds (both contain mostly omega 9), and coconut oil (mostly saturated). Despite negative press, the saturated fat in coconut oil is not harmful to heart health. In fact it has been shown to not affect LDL ("bad" cholesterol) and to raise HDL cholesterol ("good" cholesterol) which forms a more beneficial ratio of LDL to HDL. Most scientists and doctors will agree that the LDL to HDL ratio is one of the most important heart disease markers available.

Coconut oil has also been shown to beneficially shrink waist circumferences in women when compared to soybean oil. [8] Saturated fats in general have been unfairly vilified over the past several decades. Information on this topic, and for example why most (but not all) types of red meat are not bad for your heart at all, can be found in the free report at nutrientbalance.com/dietsodareport.

Coconut oil, almonds/almond oil, and olive oil have not been studied internally in relation to growing hair. However, in topical usage, coconut oil has been proven to actually penetrate the hair root while other oils were unable. In addition, topical coconut oil, when used before or after shampooing, was shown to reduce hair protein loss and to be beneficial in preventing hair damage. [9] More on topical coconut oil will be included in the final section on other therapies.

In addition, if you look at the same study I quoted previously regarding fatty acids and the conversion of testosterone to DHT, you will find that oleic acid which is found in almonds and olive oil, and lauric acid which is found in coconut oil, are included on the list of inhibitory fatty acids. This indicates that almonds, olive oil, and coconut oil also help normalize DHT levels. [34]

My own personal experience with coconut oil taken orally (a tablespoonful or two per day) has appeared to be very beneficial in preventing hair loss and potentially promoting hair growth. Several times, I have run out of coconut oil, and each time within a couple of days my hair began to feel straw-like and started to appear all over the shoulders of my shirts. After reintroducing the oil each time, the straw-like effect and the hair fall-out mostly went away. You can guess that I buy coconut oil well in advance now, so that I don't ever run out.

Initially in experimenting with olive oil and almonds, I didn't notice the same beneficial effects as with the coconut oil. However, I believe this was due to the fact that I had already been consuming a significant amount of each. There was one week in which I realized I had not consumed much olive oil or any almonds. By the end of the week, my hair was thinning noticeably and falling out fairly fast considering I mostly had it under control otherwise. When I reintroduced the almonds and olive oil to previous levels, my hair regained its thickness and much, much less fell out within about two or three days.

Silica

One mineral that is largely overlooked in human health is silica or silicon (this is a natural mineral, and *not* silicone with an "e" at the end, which is the synthetic version made famous by breast implants). Mostly if you look up silica on the internet or elsewhere, you will find warnings that it is harmful to respiratory health in the form of silica dust which is found in many factory and mining situations. This is true; however, it is also true that humans need silica in their diet, as it is crucial for five areas: bone, joint, skin, nail, and hair health.

The media largely discusses calcium as the bone-building mineral, and it is true that calcium plays a huge part in bone-building and other body processes.

However, what they fail to realize is that the calcium in bones only hardens with a proper amount of silica. Bone is also largely built due to the effects of estrogen and testosterone. This is why osteoporosis is often seen in post-menopausal women.

In a study on rats with ovaries removed in order to reduce estrogen and therefore cause a state of osteopenia (the precursor to osteoporosis), two groups were fed diets with or without silicon added. In the silicon group, not only did the rats not lose bone mass, they actually gained bone mass. In the non-silicon group, the rats lost bone mass as expected. [10]

While this is not a book about bones or osteoporosis, you can see that perhaps silicon is a mineral that people have been overlooking for general health.

Now back to the hair issue. There is a type of silica supplement called choline-stabilized orthosilicic acid that comes in pill or drop form. Researchers at the University of Cincinnati did a study on supplementing this form of silica for the purpose of hair health in women. At the end of the study, it was concluded that supplementing with this form of silica was beneficial in strengthening and thickening the hair when compared to the placebo. [11]

Does strengthening and thickening of hair mean that it will also not fall out or grow back in places that it no longer exists? This much was not studied. However, I would venture to guess that at least hair fall-out would be reduced with thicker hair, because thicker hair sits more firmly in the follicle.

The type of silica studied is sold in stores as the brand Biosil, and a few other brand names. Other types of silica supplements may or may not work as well. I personally have taken an herb called horsetail with a standardized amount of silica and I have noticed at least modest benefits in terms of thicker and smoother hair that falls out less. The choline-stabilized orthosilicic acid forms are much more expensive than standardized horsetail, and it might (or might not) work better than the kind I use. What I can say is that there are far more testimonials for the orthosilicic acid forms than the horsetail forms, but this could also mean that simply more people bought it.

Iron

Before discussing iron, I should note that high iron levels are potentially even more harmful than low. Low iron leads to anemia and other symptoms like hair loss, while too much can increase heart disease and cancer risk. This means that before taking iron, it is important to check your serum iron and ferritin, total iron binding capacity, and transferrin saturation.

Serum ferritin is the test you want to most closely monitor, because it indicates whole body iron stores and it is the marker that correlates with hair loss according to the Journal of Investigative Dermatology. [12] However, you should discuss iron findings with your doctor because various combinations of low, normal, and high readings on all four tests are indicative of various conditions.

If ferritin levels are on the low side (under 30 ng/mL), while the other markers are in the normal ranges, both men and women should supplement and check levels. Test regularly and stop supplementing when levels reach 60 ng/mL because high iron is risky and does not help hair loss more than normal levels. Try to stay between 40 ng/mL and 60 ng/mL.

According to conventional medicine experts, iron deficiency is almost never a problem in men and in post-menopausal women because it is the loss of blood in the menstrual cycle or in pregnancy that leads to low iron levels. However, I have seen plenty of cases of men and post-menopausal women with low serum ferritin. In my own case, when I don't supplement with iron, I see ferritin levels drop to the low side of the scale, and you can be assured that I am not menstruating.

I believe that most types of iron supplements are sufficient to restore ferritin levels. In my own experience, my levels were restored simply by using a multi-vitamin containing 18 mg iron, though menstruating women may find they need more. I'm not sure how well iron worked for my own hair loss, because other therapies in this book had already helped. However, I do think my hair seems much smoother and softer, in a good way, when on iron.

For those with very serious iron deficiency, meaning ferritin below 15 ng/mL and certainly below 10 ng/mL, more iron should be taken daily than 18 mg. Take around 50 mg and keep testing every month or two to get your dose correct. Doctors may also prescribe high doses.

2. THYROID HEALTH

One significant cause of hair loss is thyroid imbalance, and correcting the issue should help hair health if this is one of the causes. For a bit of background, the thyroid gland is located in the front of the neck near the Adam's apple in men, or where the Adam's apple would be in women. The main purpose of the thyroid is to regulate metabolism, or the rate at which you burn calories throughout the day.

Those who have an under-active thyroid or who have low thyroid hormone levels are hypothyroid and generally burn calories too slowly, causing an increase in weight and a decrease in energy. Those who have an overactive thyroid or high thyroid hormone levels are hyperthyroid; they burn calories too quickly and often have an excess of energy, at least temporarily.

In addition to calorie burning and metabolic issues, thyroid imbalance can also cause other symptoms, namely cold sensitivity, depression, fatigue, dry skin, weight gain, and *thin, brittle hair* and nails. [13]

Thyroid hormones are created by three compounds found in the diet: iodine, selenium, and tyrosine. The first two are minerals, while tyrosine is an amino acid (amino acids are the building blocks of all proteins). Paying attention to consuming and absorbing enough protein, as mentioned in the first section on dietary deficiencies, should ensure that you get enough tyrosine.

Bigger concerns are related to iodine and selenium. First, to get enough selenium, I simply recommend that you take a multivitamin that contains at least 100% of the RDA of selenium. 200% would be a little better, but don't go too high, because selenium toxicity exists in addition to deficiency. You wouldn't ever reach toxicity by taking 200% of the RDA of selenium along with a general diet.

Next, we need to discuss iodine. This is a tricky subject, because many health practitioners have vastly different ideas about what a healthy amount of iodine should be. Iodine is not largely found in the diet, except in the form of iodized salt and in various types of seaweed, which most people don't eat. A moderate amount is found in milk and cod fish, and a small amount is found in other dairy and animal products. However, if you don't have much salt during the day, or if your salt is not iodized (often sea salt and other healthier varieties of salt are not iodized), you risk running a deficiency. Therefore, you should consider supplementing iodine.

The RDA for iodine is only 150 micrograms (mcg) and most multivitamins contain this amount. However, there is a lot of dissent in the medical community as to whether this small of an amount is really enough to keep the thyroid supplied with enough raw materials to make thyroid hormones, when many other areas of the body also make use of the mineral.

Because this is such a controversial area, and because the scientific literature itself is not complete enough to accurately light the path toward the truth, I will play the middle ground here for the purpose of improving your thyroid health. First, have thyroid labs tested, including total and free T3 and T4, as well as TSH. Also ask to have thyroid antibodies tested (when positive these often indicate Hashimoto's thyroiditis, an autoimmune thyroid disorder). The antibodies to test are anti-thyroid peroxidase antibody (anti-TPO) and sometimes antithyroglobulin antibody as well (some doctors prefer to only test the first)..

If either of these antibodies come up positive (indicating possible Hashimoto's or Graves Disease), be careful about supplementing iodine. In this case, it is probably best to not take more iodine than is in your multi vitamin and in your general diet. This is because an overabundance of iodine can actually worsen Hashimoto's thyroiditis.

If these tests come up negative, and your other hormone levels (T3/T4) read normal, low-normal, or low - but not high-normal or high - then it is probably a good idea to supplement a little more iodine than the RDA. (A *high* TSH is likely indicative of hypothyroidism). I believe a good amount is around 1,100 micrograms (note that this is *micrograms or mcg*, not milligrams or mg, a VERY important distinction because milligrams would be far too much), which is the US government's tolerable upper intake. This means it is the highest amount an average person should consume on a daily basis while having little or no risk of adverse effects.

Keep in mind also that many highly respected physicians recommend iodine in amounts of 12.5 mg up to 50mg and sometimes even more (this is equal to 12,500 to 50,000 micrograms or mcg). They generally report few, if any, side effects. However, for the purpose of this book, I won't recommend higher than the tolerable upper intake. If you are interested in going higher than this amount, it is a good idea to see a doctor first. Actually, if you suspect a thyroid issue in general, it is a good idea to see a doctor to get tested.

So, which iodine is good to take? I recommend a brand known as Iosol. This comes in drops and one drop is equal to 1,830 mcg. While this is a little higher than the 1,100 mcg per day, you can take one drop around 2 to 3 days on and one day off in a cycle fashion in order to achieve close to the 1,100 mcg average amount. One small bottle of this is inexpensive and will last a very long time when only taking a drop or so per day.

My own experience was that Iosol did in fact contribute to better looking and healthier hair (I use an average of three drops a day, but again consult a doctor before adding more than I recommended above). Iodine is likely to help your hair if you experience at least a few of the other symptoms of thyroid disorder such as cold hands, fatigue, etc. If you find that it doesn't help, then it is probably the case that you either weren't iodine deficient in the first place, or you need even more iodine than the amount recommended. A good way to assess this is to look at a list of hypothyroid symptoms, and speak with a natural-minded doctor (ACAM.org is a good place to search for this type of doctor) in regards to testing thyroid and iodine sufficiency.

3. PROSTATE HEALTH

(Women can feel free to skip this chapter and move on to chapter four, regarding calcification. All recommendations in the other chapters do pertain to women, and every recommendation in the book is applicable to men).

If you have done a significant amount of research on male pattern baldness, you probably already found that DHT is a hormone implicated in both benign prostate hyperplasia or BPH (the common non-cancerous prostate growth condition), and in hair loss. You probably also recall DHT from the section above on fatty acids. DHT stands for dihydro-testosterone, and is created from testosterone in a reaction catalyzed by the enzyme 5-Alpha-Reductase (5-AR). Yes, a lot of big words here, but you should know that 5-AR inhibitors are the types of therapies that you should use to lower DHT if necessary. 5-AR inhibitors can be drugs, foods, or supplements.

Finesteride, also known as Propecia, is one such 5-AR inhibiting drug that is FDA approved to both treat BPH and reduce hair loss. I don't recommend this drug based on the significant risk for long term and possibly permanent sexual dysfunction, after the medication is discontinued. [14] Instead, see the therapies below.

Just because you have hair loss does not mean that you necessarily have DHT levels that are outside the normal range. It would be a wise idea to get your DHT tested, because if it is normal, low-normal, or low, than you shouldn't use any of the therapies in this section, aside from the essential fatty acids. If it is high-normal or high, it is probably a good idea to use some of the therapies, at least for a short time. Most doctors would be willing to write an order for this test, but if not, you can go through directlabs.com to order the test without a prescription. This test costs a moderate amount of money, but it is worth it to know what you are really dealing with.

I mentioned above that essential fatty acids, omega 3 and omega 6, along with oleic acid (almonds/olive oil), lauric acid (coconut oil), and GLA (evening primrose, borage, or black currant seed oil) are among the best ways to reduce DHT levels. It could even be argued that a deficiency of these oils is the reason the DHT is elevated in the first place. That statement may or may not be true, but it is true that raising intake of these fatty acids in the amounts I listed in the nutrient deficiency section of this book (above) is both beneficial for your hair, your prostate, and your overall health. Please reread that section if you forgot about it.

Saw Palmetto

The first herb to mention when it comes to reducing DHT levels is saw palmetto. This is the most well known herb for prostate health, although not necessarily the best. Studies do indicate that it is a potent 5-AR inhibitor. [15] Most herbs have a compound or mineral that is an active ingredient and in the case of saw palmetto, the main active ingredient is beta sitosterol. Beta sitosterol has also been proven to lower cholesterol, and is often added to margarines and spreads (which I don't recommend eating) so that the companies can make the FDA-approved claim that the spread reduces cholesterol.

Some experts recommend beta sitosterol taken as a supplement in place of saw palmetto because they say it is more potent. From my medical literature research, I found that studies on saw palmetto and beta sitosterol appear to get similar results in regards to prostate health. If you get saw palmetto, be sure to find a product standardized to 85% or more fatty acids and sterols.

Black Tea

Another interesting option to try, although not scientifically verified, is black tea. Studies on mice found that while on black tea, they showed a 72% drop in DHT levels and increased testosterone by 34.4%. [16]

Certainly, studies would have to be repeated on mice, and tried on humans before one could definitively say that black tea lowers DHT levels in humans. However, 72% is a promising number, and as a medicinal ingredient, it doesn't get too much safer than black tea.

Of course you can drink several cups of black tea throughout the day, but you can also purchase black tea extract pills. It appears likely that the compound most beneficial to health in black tea (found in higher levels than in green tea) is theaflavin. Look for a black tea extract with a standardized amount of theaflavin, and take the amount recommended on the package. I have not yet tried this therapy, so unfortunately, I can't offer you my personal experience regarding hair health.

Prostate Massage

Caution: The following therapy is recommended for those with chronic prostatitis, BPH (enlarged prostate), and those without prostate issues, but is *NOT* indicated for prostate cancer or acute prostatitis due to potential for spread of infection or cancer.

If you have experienced any amount of prostate symptoms or enlargement in addition to your hair loss, I recommend using an in-home prostate massager. This is a device made out of FDA-approved plastic and inserted into the rectum so that it can press down against the prostate. To see an example, go to www.highisland.com. These have not been studied in relation to hair loss, but a preliminary study showed that they have very significant and beneficial effects for prostate health, both for chronic prostatitis (an inflammatory and/or infectious prostate condition) and for benign prostate hyperplasia (BPH). 92.2% of BPH patients found at least some improvement using the device, and 88% of prostatitis patients saw at least some improvement. [17]

I personally have experienced chronic prostatitis, and have seen a dramatic, though not permanent, reduction in pain immediately following usage of the prostate massage device. In addition, it appears to me that the massage sessions have been very beneficial for hair health as well. Less falls out, and hair seems to thicken up within a day or two. An internet search also reveals a few other guys who have had this positive experience with hair, and dozens who have had positive experiences for their prostate health.

Even for those with no prostate issues, the device could likely act as a preventative for future prostate problems, which most men end up having eventually. In addition, it could possibly be an immediate help for hair (although evidence for hair is anecdotal at this point).

If it is true that the prostate massager works for hair loss, it probably would be based on the same principle of prostate and hair health both being tied to the conversion from testosterone to DHT. The preliminary study on prostate massage was very successful for prostate health in terms of pain symptoms, urinary flow, and overall quality of life, but it didn't address DHT levels or hair health specifically. Hopefully at some point soon, these areas will be addressed and perhaps confirmed.

Be sure to follow the instructions given at www.highisland.com/pm_instructions.php. Also, be sure to clean before and after use each time, and use plenty of lubrication. You can buy lubrication at the same time as the device. However, for a natural option, the company Good Clean Love offers an organic and effective lubricant.

A good device to start with is the PS-2 because it is small and easiest to use. If your main concern is hair health, and not prostate health additionally, you will never need another device. If you also have BPH or prostatitis, you might want to later try one of the other models to see if you can get even better results.

4. CALCIFICATION

The next pressing issue to be aware of when hair health is a concern is calcification, or the process of calcium hardening in soft tissues rather than staying where it is supposed to be, which is in the bones and flowing in the blood stream. Calcification is present in many disease processes, including calcium build up in the sides of arteries to cause heart disease, in the joints to cause arthritis, in the brain to cause Alzheimer's, in the kidneys to cause kidney stones, in the urinary tract to cause prostatitis or cystitis, and in many other regions.

One potentially calcified region that you should be aware of is your scalp. A gross anatomy technician serving at the University of Illinois School of Medicine from 1916 to 1917 had the job of removing cadaver brains from the rest of the body in order to store them in the neurology classes (definitely "gross" anatomy, if you will). In the process of removing the brains, he made the observation, and reported it to the Journal of the American Medical Association, that those cadavers of bald people showed significant calcification in the skull bones that "firmly knitted the cranial sutures." In contrast, calcification was not seen in those bodies that still had a full head of hair. [18]

Therefore it would make sense that natural therapies aimed at clearing out calcium deposits should work at least to some degree in loosening up calcium in the skull and allowing hair to once again grow freely. The following two methods, IP-6 and vitamin K2, have not yet been studied for hair health, but they are the best choices for elimination of general calcification.

IP6

What is IP6? Another name for IP6 is phytate or phytic acid. Phytates are compounds found largely in whole grains and in seeds. They are the major food storage site of phosphorus. However, some health experts argue that eating foods containing phytates makes those foods not as healthy as they should be. This is because the phytates bind with healthy minerals and therefore don't allow their absorption into the body. So, if a piece of whole wheat bread has magnesium in it, but it also has phytates, you are absorbing less than the full amount of magnesium because it is bound up to the phytate and passes out of the body, unabsorbed.

Therefore, there is a point to the fact that phytates are sometimes not ideal for health. However, I would never recommend consuming refined grains (white bread or white pasta) instead of the whole grain counterparts, because the refined versions don't even have the minerals to begin with. At least with whole grains, you are getting some of the minerals.

IP6 comes in a capsule form that people take as a dietary supplement. But wait... you say to yourself. You just told me phytates aren't good because they don't allow for mineral absorption. Well yes, but when you take them in supplement form (and even in food form), they are exceptionally healthy in other ways- here's why...

First, IP6 is known to be a cancer fighting nutrient. In fact, it is much better known for this quality than for its calcification-clearing effects. IP6 has been found to differentiate malignant cancer cells, which means it helps them revert to normal cells. It also enhances the effects of general chemotherapy, helps to stop metastasis (cancer spreading to other regions), and improves the quality of life for cancer patients. [19]

When various natural therapies are good for cancer treatment, this almost always means that they are also a cancer preventative, and this is very true in the case of IP6.

Okay, but this is not a cancer book, and you are interested in hair. When you take IP6 in supplement form, your job is to separate it from all other food, drugs, or supplements by at least an hour both before and after. The reason you should do this is because IP6 latches on to minerals most vigorously when they haven't yet been absorbed or digested, or when they are in places they are not supposed to be. So when there are no minerals to bind to because nothing recently has been eaten, the only thing around that IP6 can latch onto is excess or free calcium and iron.

As we saw above, it has been observed that calcification in the skull is correlated strongly to baldness, so if IP6 can clear out this calcification, all the better. I also mentioned that it clears out iron, which also probably contributes to its anti-cancer effects (iron that is not bound up in red blood cells can feed cancer cells and pathogens). Here are a few studies that verify IP6's ability to clear out calcification and free iron. [20] [21]

Does IP-6 help with hair loss? As noted, no direct studies have been done, however in my own case, there did seem to be a modest improvement in hair loss and hair re-growth. As with any other therapy in this book, it is not a solo therapy, but in combination with a few to several other therapies, it should be of significant benefit.

Vitamin K2

Vitamin K might be the least well-known vitamin. It is best known for its blood clotting properties. In fact, the clot preventing drug called coumadin is a vitamin K antagonist, meaning it stops the clotting action of vitamin K.

When speaking of blood clotting, it is important to note that this is a property mainly of vitamin K1. There are two types of vitamin K found in the body: vitamin K1 and K2. A third type (K3) has been synthesized. The synthetic version (K3) is neither healthy nor safe, so there is no need to concern yourself with it.

Vitamin K1 is mostly found in green vegetables and a few veggies of other colors. Vitamin K2 is not largely found in the diet except for a small amount in various meats, dairy, and eggs, and a large amount in nattokinase, which is a fermented soy food consumed more so in Asian countries. K2 is also synthesized from K1 in the intestines. However, even if one's intestines are working perfectly well, it can be argued that not enough K2 becomes available for optimal health.

In contrast to K1, Vitamin K2's main function is related to its calcium regulation. Similar to IP6, it prevents calcification, [22] but in addition to this, it also promotes the formation of bone material, so it helps to protect against bone loss and osteoporosis. [23]

After taking vitamin K2, in contrast to IP-6, I did not notice too much of an effect on my own hair. However, based on the extensive studies of its other health promoting abilities, I still take it, and I recommend it is worth a shot for others to try for hair health. Many more significant benefits of vitamin K2 are outlined in my free report, "Diet Soda Makes You Fatter Than Regular and 10 More Shocking Health Truths." This can be downloaded at nutrientbalance.com/dietsodareport.

5. OTHER THERAPIES

Essential Oils

I didn't mention above that there are several types of alopecia, which is the scientific term for hair loss. Androgenic alopecia is usually found in males and is related to DHT levels, as mentioned above. Alopecia arreta is the loss of hair in patches, which is often caused by an autoimmune condition. [24] Traction alopecia is caused by ponytails, braids, hair relaxer solutions, and hot irons (you may want to lessen or stop usage of any of those, if necessary, to see if they are causing a problem). Lastly, alopecia totalis relates to hair loss over the whole head, while alopecia universalis involves hair loss over the whole body.

Regarding alopecia arreata, I believe that it would be the case that several of the therapies listed in the other sections would help for this potentially autoimmune condition. However, one natural therapy has been studied specifically for alopecia arreata with promising results. It is the topical application of various essential oils.

Before I begin, let me clear up some confusion: essential oils and essential fatty acids are not the same thing. Essential fatty acids refers to omega 3 and omega 6 dietary oils that we discussed before. Essential oils refers to various medicinal oils that are usually quite potent, have a strong aroma, and are derived from herbs and other plants. A few examples are thyme, rosemary, lavender, and cedarwood oils. In fact, these four oils were studied together in a trial reported in the Archives of Dermatology.

The trial split 86 alopecia arreata patients into two groups. One group put jojoba oil (a common dilutor oil) and grapeseed oil (a common dietary oil) on their hair. The others put the same two oils on, but their solution also contained the four essential oils (thyme, rosemary, lavender, and cedarwood oils). According to "blinded" observers viewing pictures of the results, (blinded means they didn't know to which group the photos belonged), 44% of the essential oil group showed improvement in hair growth, whereas only 15% of the control group showed improvement.

According to the study, patients were to massage the oils into their scalps for 2 full minutes each night. The jojoba oil was 3 ml (about half a teaspoon), the grapeseed oil was 20 ml (about 4 teaspoons), and there were two drops of thyme, three drops of lavender, three drops of rosemary, and two drops of cedarwood oils. In order to perform the massage, take each of these ingredients, mix them up well, and apply to the full area of the scalp, especially concentrating on areas where hair is lacking. After the two minute oil massage, a warm towel should be wrapped around the head to help absorption.

There was one man in this trial who also had androgenic (DHT-related) hair loss, and it was noted that the oils appeared to help moderately in his case as well. If you follow the link to the study, you will see a picture of a different man with stunning regrowth of hair. He was almost completely bald at the trial's start and had close to a full head of hair after seven months. [25]

I should note that a few years ago, there were studies on a few boys who had been using bath products made of lavender, and they experienced estrogenic effects in the body, such as small amounts of breast growth. After discontinuing the products, the effect went away. There was some dissent as to whether this was truly the effect of the lavender or something else. However, to be on the safe side, men especially may want to avoid the lavender, and instead use the other three oils. On the other hand, lavender has also shown activity against DHT, [26] and this may be part of the reason the therapy works so well. So perhaps using a smaller amount of lavender, or more sporadic usage, would allow for the benefits without the side effects.

Regarding purchasing oils, look for brands that contain only 100% pure oil. Now Foods, Aura Casia, and Young Living all sell quality oils. Small bottles are usually inexpensive, and when using only a few drops at a time, they last a while. But *be careful*, because essential oils are very strong and can burn the skin, eyes, or mouth, etc. when not diluted properly. Please use as directed in this chapter, or as directed by an aromatherapy professional. Follow directions closely, because a wrong ratio of ingredients could lead to negative effects. If you have any adverse effects by using the oils, try to instead use only one to three of them, rather than all four. Rosemary is the oil that is most widely regarded for its hair-enhancing properties, so try it first if you are only using one. Then add or switch oils depending on the outcome.

Shampoo Recommendation

Some people ask if there is a certain type of shampoo to buy for the purpose of re-growing hair. Research is generally lacking in this area, and I have found that most shampoos that claim to be beneficial for hair loss actually have only poor to moderate testimonials, indicating that benefits are probably non-existent or placebo related.

This being said, I do have a shampoo that I recommend. It does not claim to be a "hair-loss" shampoo, but it contains ingredients that have been verified by research to be healthy for hair growth when topically applied. This shampoo is called "Dr. Bronner's Magic Soap: Peppermint Pure Castile Soap."

The main ingredient in this shampoo, following water, is saponified (or soap-like) coconut oil. Recall from the discussion in the first section that topically-applied coconut oil is the only scientifically verified oil to penetrate the scalp and protect against hair protein loss and related damage. [9]

Of course, you could use straight coconut oil, but at room temperature, the oil is a solid, and therefore you would have to heat it or rub it between your hands for a while in order for it to become a liquid which would therefore be spreadable around your scalp. The coconut oil in Dr. Bronner's shampoo is already liquefied and also is not in a greasy oil format, but in a soap-like state. This makes it very simple to experience the scientifically proven benefits of coconut oil.

Another key ingredient in Dr. Bronner's shampoo is jojoba oil. Recall that in the study done on the essential oils, the carrier oil for both groups was jojoba oil. While those in the group with only jojoba and grapeseed oils improved hair health significantly less than those in the group that also had essential oils, it should be noted that even the carrier oil-only group saw a 15% improvement in hair. It is possible that this amount is scientifically insignificant. However, keep in mind that the observers were from a third party and had no interest in whether the study participants had hair growth. Therefore, it was impossible to have a placebo effect. My point in all of this is that jojoba oil with grapeseed oil likely had a small but important positive effect on hair. Grapeseed oil is not included in Dr. Bronner's shampoo, but other oils, such as olive and hemp seed, are included, which may or may not have hair growth benefits as well.

Lastly, I should note that it is possible to do a modified version of the essential oil protocol (described above) using your shampoo rather than an oil massage, which could get messy. Of course, it is possible that this method might not work as well as the researched method, but I believe that it is close enough that there should be significant benefits with less work.

The method is as follows: Take the thyme, cedarwood, rosemary, and lavender oil bottles into the shower. Remember that the study used 4.5 teaspoons of combined jojoba and grapeseed oils, and had 2 to 3 drops of each of the oils put in the mix. You should try to keep that ratio similar, but at around half the amount of everything, because 4.5 teaspoons of shampoo would be too much.

Therefore, pour approximately 2 teaspoons of shampoo (don't skimp because you need proper dilution ratios for the oils) followed by the 1 drop each of thyme and cedarwood oils, and 2 drops each of rosemary and lavender oils (not quite half, but it is impossible to have half of 3 drops). Stir up the mixture with the opposite hand enough so that everything appears mixed together very thoroughly.

Similar to the method in the study, make sure that you shampoo all areas of your scalp, getting underneath the hair, and focusing the most on areas where hair loss is most prominent. Let the shampoo and oils sit on your head for two minutes. It is difficult to do this if you are just sitting there, so it is a good idea to plan to wash the rest of your body while the shampoo sits on your scalp. You are now double-tasking in the shower... your boss would be proud.

Grapeseed Extract

Researchers in Japan embarked upon a mission in the late 1990s: take hundreds of plant compounds and determine which of them could be used for the purposes of re-growing hair. About 1000 compounds were examined in total, and in the end, the one that stuck out was proanthocyanidins (sounds just how you would read it). These are specialized antioxidant molecules found largely in grape seed and pine bark extracts.

When applied topically to shaven mice, researchers found that those mice that received the active proanthocyanidins grew hair back at a rate of 230% that of controls. I am a little confused as to why the researchers linked shaven mice with balding men and women, because it seems like these are two very different processes. However, despite this difference, researchers thought the research was enough to conclude that topical grape seed proanthocyanidins are a possibility for the treatment of hair loss. [27]

In a second study by the same researchers, they concluded that proanthocyanidin B-2, B-3, and C-1, (three different varieties), all showed significant hair growth effects in mice, as well as in vitro (in a test tube). [28]

Not many companies offer products including topical proanthocyanidins. However, one lotion that is available is called Crinagen. Unfortunately, I was unable to find any reviews or testimonials on the product except for one from a man who was disappointed that it was overly sticky and hard to manage in his hair. He was unaware if there were benefits because he stopped it shortly after starting. On the Crinagen website, there is one before and after picture of a Crinagen user, but the before picture is quite blurry, so it is hard to tell if there were any benefits at all.

I have not tried any topical application of proanthocyanidins, however I have taken grape seed extract capsules internally. I was hoping that there would be a correlation and that the capsules would also do positive things for the hair. After several months, this didn't appear to be the case, or at least not for me. However, internal proanthocyanidins have been studied for several other health improvement areas, and it looks like they hold promise for lowering blood pressure and cholesterol, reducing edema and venous insufficiency, and preventing various cancers. [29]

Regarding topical usage of proanthocyanadins, I don't have a recommendation at this time, although you could try Crinagen if so inclined. I have thought about ways to create your own topical application, but I'm unsure of how to do so properly. Grape seed oil (as mentioned in the essential oil study above as a carrier oil), does not contain any proanthocyanadins according to researchers. [30]

A grape seed extract capsule could be opened and poured into shampoo, but I doubt this would have the correct properties to penetrate the scalp. Unfortunately, for now it looks like proanthocyanadins are not a viable option.

Panax Ginseng

Another promising topical compound is panax ginseng. Panax is the Asian variety of Ginseng. There are also American and Korean ginseng varieties, among others. Panax ginseng extract was found to possess hair growth promotion abilities in a mouse model, which scientists attributed to compounds called saponins. [31]

A second study examining the effects of fructus panax ginseng (a different variety of Asian panax ginseng), also found that the compound has the potential to become a treatment for hair regeneration based on its effects on mice. In this study, the fructus form was found to significantly enhance anagen times, which means the time that hair can grow and mature in the root. [32]

It should also be noted here that hairless mice may or may not correlate with hair loss in men or women in regards to using the same treatment. However, in contrast to the grape seed treatment (above), panax ginseng is available in several topical hair products, including lotions, shampoos, and conditioners. A search online for testimonials through Amazon.com and iherb.com showed that a significant number of men and women were happy with these products in regards to hair growth and thickening potential. I haven't tried this option, so unfortunately I cannot weigh in with my own experience. See the action guide (chapter six) for suggestions of a few brand names that have natural ingredients and have achieved positive testimonials.

Vitamin E Tocotrienols

Most people are aware that there are several types of B vitamins, including B1, B2, folic acid, and many more. However, most people are unaware that there are eight types of E vitamins. This is because the vast majority of multivitamins and vitamin E supplements contain only one type of vitamin E: alpha tocopherol. There are actually four types of tocopherols: the alpha, beta, gamma, and delta fractions. Alpha and gamma tocopherol are found most widely in the diet.

In addition to the tocopherols, there are also four tocotrienols, which similarly have the fractions alpha, beta, delta, and gamma. Scientists initially ignored the tocotrienols, because they are not widely found in foods, and because they are not essential to health. Recall that "essential" in health terms means that you must obtain it from the diet or supplements or you will become deficient, leading to a decline in health.

While people could live a long healthy life without ever touching a tocotrienol version of vitamin E, it could be argued that they couldn't get to the pinnacle of good health without them. In other words, tocotrienols might be essential to "optimal health" as opposed to just "health."

The reason I make this claim is based on the research piling up only within the last decade regarding the health benefits of vitamin E tocotrienols. It appears that tocotrienols are likely to help lower heart disease risk, [33] improve insulin sensitivity, thereby lowering diabetes risk, [34] work synergistically with chemotherapy against breast cancer and lower chemotherapy's side effects, [35] help fight against prostate cancer, and much more.

Tocotrienols have also been reported to help re-grow hair in the case of androgenic alopecia. According to a study from the University of Science in Malaysia, after eight months of taking tocotrienols, participants saw a 34.5% increase in actual hair count in a specific section of hair. Those taking the placebo had a 0.1% decrease in hair count. Researchers concluded that it was likely the antioxidant effect in the scalp creating the positive outcome. [36]

When trying this myself, I didn't note the same results. However, I might not have given the therapy adequate time to work. The study noted about half of the results were achieved after four months and the other half were achieved after eight months. Most of the other therapies I have noted in this book seemed to take effect within a couple weeks, and many of them within days. So after around a month, I didn't see or feel any hair benefit, and this may have been unfair.

Surprisingly, I did find a very significant and lasting reduction in prostate pain (from chronic prostatitis) by taking the tocotrienols, which is the main reason I continue to take it, along with its general health promotion and disease preventative benefits. This pain reduction is interesting based on the significant ties between prostate and hair health as noted earlier.

A search for testimonials on tocotrienols and hair health doesn't reveal too many positive results. However, it is possible that, like me, most others gave a few weeks or a month to assess results while results are really only possible after four to eight months or more, as indicated in the research.

Laser Treatment

I would hope at this point, with all of the above recommendations, that you will be able to find diet and supplemental changes that mostly or completely fix your issue with hair loss. If this is not the case, there are a few more non-drug options. The first is laser treatment. This is available both at clinics (possibly at one near you), or by using a purchased home device.

Probably the most well known home unit is the HairMax Laser Comb. According to a study on 110 male patients in Florida and reported in Pubmed, the LaserComb did show a significant amount of hair re-growth after a six month period when compared to a sham device (placebo). [37] After researching the internet for reviews, it doesn't appear that the LaserComb is as well thought of as the study would have you believe. But again, this could be the case where people need to wait six months to make an assessment, and they only gave it a month or two, for example. I haven't personally tried the laser comb, as the sum of the other therapies at this point seems to keep me with a full head of hair. However, if at some point I try it, I will update this book.

Toppik

If you have tried everything, and still can't get your hair to grow as you would like, there is one solution short of a toupee, plugs, transplant, or drugs. It is called Toppik. Toppik is a powder that is made out of keratin protein (the same protein your own hair is made of), as well as various vitamins. You sprinkle on the powder in the fashion directed by the package, and the powder begins to fuse with your existing hair, creating fuller, thicker hair that covers up minor bald spots nicely. Toppik works on areas of thinning hair, but not on areas that are completely bald.

Toppik is rated very well in regards to how it looks and feels. Most people say that it is impossible to tell that Toppik powder is not actually your real hair. A few have complained that the powder can get on a pillow or forehead, but others say that it is easy to learn how to avoid this situation.

Some people might say that using Toppik is "cheating" because it is not actually your real hair, and because it will wash off in the shower. In a sense this is true, but some men and women are to the point where no treatment, even drugs, will help. Toppik can help in this scenario. In addition, for those who are trying out the natural treatments listed in this book, Toppik can be a temporary solution to tide you over. Because it washes out, you can always remove it and assess progress for the natural therapies that are hopefully growing your true hair back.

6. ACTION GUIDE

At this point you have read all of the therapies that I have made available. I will now make a list with a set of category ratings so that you can assess for yourself if it is worth it to try one therapy over another. The criteria will be as follows:

Scientific evidence - More than one human trial with positive results would get five stars. A single positive human study gets four stars. An animal trial with theoretical basis gets three stars. An in-vitro study (test tube) with a theoretical basis, or a human study that is only indirectly related to hair loss, gets two stars. No solid scientific evidence gets a single star.

Web Testimonials - Lots of positive user experience documented on the web gets five stars, where few if any web reviews gets one star.

My Own (Author's) Experience - If the therapy was noticeably positive over time, this gets four to five stars. If I didn't notice a change, it gets one star. Small amount of positive change would be a two star and so forth.

Expense - In this case, a lower cost is better, so I give low cost items five stars and expensive items one star, etc.

Other Positive Health Effects - In some cases, therapies are worth a try simply because they are healthy in ways other than hair growth. Good examples of this are vitamin E tocotrienols and vitamin K2.

Method - This is exactly how to go about doing the therapy including possible brands and dosages.

THERAPY LIST

Optimizing Protein Intake / Hemp Protein

Scientific Evidence - Four Stars (Strong evidence although most people are already sufficient and therefore it wouldn't help them improve hair further, except possibly with hemp protein).

Web Testimonials - One Star for general protein consumption, Two Stars for Hemp Protein powder

Author's Experience - Two Stars for general protein, Four Stars for Hemp Protein powder (which contains minerals, fiber, and fatty acids).

Expense - Five Stars for general protein consumption, Four Stars for Hemp Protein powder

Other Positive Health Effects - Five Stars

Method - Take your weight in pounds and divide by 2.2. This new number is your weight in kilograms. Take your kilogram weight and multiply by 1.2 if you are sedentary, 1.5 if you are active or if you have a chronic infection or a chronic inflammatory condition, or 1.8 if you are active and also perform heavy weight bearing exercises regularly. The final number that you got is the amount in grams of protein that you should consume per day. If your digestive health is not strong, try a digestive enzyme containing at least 20,000 USP units per day. Take one pill just before or at the beginning of meals. Also, be sure to include a moderate amount of carbohydrates with protein, because carbs stimulate insulin which help carry protein to necessary areas, including the hair. Regarding hemp protein powder, take between 1 and 4 scoops per day with a carbohydrate source, for example a slice of whole wheat bread or brown rice. The scooper usually comes with the package.

Fish Oil (DHA and EPA)

Scientific Evidence - Two Stars
Web Testimonials - Two Stars
Author's Experience - Two Stars
Expense - Four Stars
Other Positive Health Effects - Five Stars
Method - Purchase fish oil soft gels. Any brand is okay so long as it says molecularly distilled. The important numbers on the label are DHA and EPA. Find out how much of DHA and EPA are in each pill (should be at least a moderate amount of each). Take enough pills so that you are consuming a total of 1200 - 2000mg per day. Some products have larger amounts of DHA or EPA per pill, such as Jarrow EPA-DHA Balance, or Natural Factors RxOmega 3 Factors. This way you only have to take 2-3 pills per day, rather than 4-6 or even more.

Omega Six Intake (Handful of Walnuts or Sunflower Seeds or Sesame / Sunflower oil)

Scientific Evidence - Two Stars
Web Testimonials - One Star
Author's Experience - Three Stars
Expense - Four Stars
Other Positive Health Effects - Five Stars
Method - Every day, make sure that you have one of the following: a large handful of raw walnuts or raw sunflower seeds, or a tablespoon or two of cold-pressed and/or virgin sunflower or sesame oil. Anything less than these amounts may cause a deficiency state to occur. Most other forms of omega 6 oils are processed or heated and therefore don't have the same positive effect in the body.

Gamma Linolenic Acid (Borage or Black Currant Seed Oil with 240mg GLA / day)

Scientific Evidence - Two Stars
Web Testimonials - Two Stars
Author's Experience - Three Stars
Expense - Four Stars
Other Positive Health Effects - Three Stars
Method - Find a borage or black currant seed oil pill that lists around 240mg of GLA on the supplement facts label per pill. Jarrow Borage GLA and Source Naturals Mega-GLA are products that fit these criteria. Take one pill per day for men, or one to two per day for women.

Omega 9 Intake

Scientific Evidence - Two Stars
Web Testimonials - One Star
Author's Experience - Three Stars
Expense - Five Stars
Other Positive Health Effects - Four Stars
Method - Simply consume at least a tablespoon of extra virgin cold pressed olive oil (great on salad), or a large handful of raw almonds per day. Consuming two or three times this amount or even more is still healthy and may help the DHT inhibition effects even more, although the calories do add up if you are watching your weight.

Coconut Oil

Scientific Evidence - Two Stars
Web Testimonials - One Star
Author's Experience - Four Stars
Expense - Four Stars
Other Positive Health Effects - Four Stars

Method - Find a brand of cold-pressed virgin or extra virgin coconut oil. Coconut oil is one of the few vegetable oils that comes as a solid. If room temperature in your kitchen is hot, keep the coconut oil in the fridge, because otherwise it will change into a liquid and go sour much more quickly. If room temperature is on the cooler side (this is usually true even with the heat on in the winter), the coconut oil will stay solid and unspoiled on the shelf. Consume a tablespoon or two of coconut oil per day, straight from the spoon (some love the taste like this and some hate it) or use it in cooking, but be sure to cook below the smoke point temperature (often listed on the bottle, but most sites say about 350 degrees).

Silica
Scientific Evidence - Four Stars
Web Testimonials - Four Stars
Author's Experience - Three Stars (Using non-studied version)
Expense - Four Stars
Other Positive Health Effects - Three Stars
Method - The scientifically studied version of silica is called choline-stabilized orthosilicic acid. This is available in the products BioSil by Natural Factors or JarrowSil by Jarrow. Note that there is a liquid form and a capsule form of these products. The liquid form is usually less than half the price per serving and has the same clinical effect. However, even the liquid form is on the expensive side. Take the amount specified on the bottle. I have found at least moderate effects using horsetail extract standardized for silica content. I use one half pill of NSI brand horsetail per day (equaling 35mg silica). Note that the study done was on women only and most web testimonials are by women. However, there is no reason

to expect different results in male hair, except that silica doesn't address the testosterone / DHA issue.

Iron

Scientific Evidence - Four Stars
Web Testimonials - Three Stars
Author's Experience - Three Stars (smoother hair)
Expense - Five Stars
Other Positive Health Effects - Three Stars
Method – Try to supplement to keep your serum ferritin levels between 40 and 60 ng/mL, but not more due to health risks. Most types of iron will work fine, including those in multi vitamins. Ferrous sulfate can upset stomach, while iron citrate, gluconate, glycinate, fumarate, and chelate are well absorbed. Depending on how low the levels are, approximately 18-50mg will work.

Iodine

Scientific Evidence - Two Stars
Web Testimonials - Three Stars
Author's Experience - Three Stars
Expense - Five Stars
Other Positive Health Effects - Four Stars
Method - The iodine I recommend is called Iosol, and it comes in liquid drop form. Simply take one drop in a glass of water and shake it up and drink. Do this two to three days on and one day off, and repeat in order to achieve the approximately 1,100mcg (remember this is micrograms or mcg, not milligrams or mg for safety's sake). You may want to consider more iodine if you think your thyroid is to blame for your hair loss. However, consult with a doctor first. If you have cold hands, dry skin, and/or weight gain as well, this is likely an indication

that the thyroid is still not healthy. Doctors that recommend taking iodine can be found at the American College for Advancement in Medicine site, (acam.org).

Saw Palmetto / Beta Sitosterol

Scientific Evidence - Four Stars

Web Testimonials - Three Stars

Author's Experience - Two Stars

Expense - Four Stars

Other Positive Health Effects - Two Stars

Method – (This recommendation is for men) There are many brands of saw palmetto and beta sitosterol. If choosing saw palmetto, be sure to pick one with 85% or higher standardized fatty acids and sterols. Either way, a good dose would be around 300mg, or as high as 600mg.

Black Tea

Scientific Evidence - Two Stars

Web Testimonials - One Star

Author's Experience - N/A

Expense - Four Stars

Other Positive Health Effects - Three Stars

Method – (This recommendation is for men) This is very vague, because no testimonials or human studies exist. However the study on mice indicating a lowering of DHT and a rise in testosterone was certain promising. It also appears that the active ingredient in black tea is theaflavins, because these are the only compounds that appears in higher quantities than in green tea, which is more known for its medicinal effects. You may try to have several cups of iced or hot black tea per day. Or what may be more efficacious and easier would be to purchase a black tea extract standardized to contain theaflavins. Two brands that make this product are Solaray and Life Extension. Take the amount recommended on the bottle.

Prostate Massage
Scientific Evidence - Two Stars
Web Testimonials - Two Stars
Author's Experience - Four Stars
Expense - Four Stars (moderate up-front expense, but minimal afterwards)
Other Positive Health Effects - Three Stars
Method – (This recommendation is for men with chronic prostatitis, BPH, or no prostate condition, but NOT for those with acute prostatitis or prostate cancer). Prostate massage devices are available for purchase at highisland.com. Purchase the PS-2 model along with lubrication from their online store. Follow directions given at their site or on the device packaging, as well as what is noted in the book in chapter 3. Performing the massage once every other day for around 15 minutes would be a good amount.

IP6
Scientific Evidence - Two Stars
Web Testimonials - One Star
Author's Experience - Three Stars
Expense - Four Stars
Other Positive Health Effects - Five Stars
Method - IP6 is taken as a pill. Start with close to 500mg total, and take it at a time at least one hour before and one hour after any other food, supplement, or drug. This will make sure that it is getting rid of calcification and free iron, rather than nutrients or drugs

that you do want. After a few days, move up to 1000mg total with the same timing. Jarrow, Source Naturals, and IP6 International have good products.

Vitamin K2
Scientific Evidence - Two Stars
Web Testimonials - One Star
Author's Experience - One Star
Expense - Four Stars
Other Positive Health Effects - Five Stars
Method - Vitamin K2 is available in a number of forms, but the kind I recommend is MK7, because it is effective and not overly expensive. I personally use the NSI brand. A good amount is between 80 and 200 mcg per day (remember again this is mcg or micrograms, not mg or milligrams - big difference).

Essential Oils (Thyme, Rosemary, Lavender, and Cedarwood)
Scientific Evidence - Four Stars
Web Testimonials - Three Stars
Author's Experience - N/A
Expense - Five Stars
Other Positive Health Effects - Two Stars
Method - Instructions were accurately explained in the two sections in the book about "Essential Oils" (page 62) and "Shampoo Recommendation" (page 66-67). Also note the cautions and purchasing info on pages 63-64.

Dr. Bronner's Magic Castile Soap Peppermint Shampoo
Scientific Evidence - Four Stars (Topical Coconut Oil study)

Web Testimonials - Two Stars
Author's Experience - Three Stars
Expense - Five Stars
Other Positive Health Effects - Two Stars
(Healthier than conventional shampoos)
Method - Purchase Dr. Bronner's Magic Castile Soap and use in the shower as shampoo. Be sure to massage the shampoo into the scalp so that it reaches all portions, and focus on areas where hair loss is most prominent. Also consider adding essential oils as described in the "Shampoo Recommendation" section of the book on pages 66-67. Please be aware of the information about purchasing oils, general oil safety, and caution for men using lavender, which are on pages 63-64.

Grape Seed Extract

Scientific Evidence - Three Stars (Topical on mice)
Web Testimonials - One Star
Author's Experience - N/A
Expense - Two Stars
Other Positive Health Effects - Three Stars
(Significant health benefits when taken internally)
Method - The study on mice was on topical application of grape seed extract proanthocyanidins. It appears that the only product available is Crinagen. You may try this (although it doesn't yet appear to have a track record of success). You may also try internal grape seed extract capsules, although this also doesn't seem to have a track record of success for hair, and didn't work in my case either. If you want to try capsules, choose those that have a standardized amount of proanthocyanidins. Olympian Labs makes a good product with 120mg grape seed extract per pill, standardized to 80:1. One or two capsules per day should be fine.

Panax Ginseng - Topical

Scientific Evidence - Three Stars

Web Testimonials - Three Stars

Author's Experience - N/A

Expense - Three Stars

Other Positive Health Effects - Two Stars

Method - There are a few companies that make topical hair products that include panax ginseng in the ingredients. Unfortunately, because shampoos are beauty products and not supplements or food, they don't need to list how much ginseng is in there. On the other hand, some of them have had decent testimonials in regards to hair growth. A few of the companies you can search for are Aubrey Organics, EO Products, and Jason Natural. Apply as directed on the package.

Vitamin E Tocotrienols

Scientific Evidence - Four Stars

Web Testimonials - Two Stars

Author's Experience - One Star (May be an unfair rating based on total time given as one month as opposed to 4 to 8)

Expense - Three Stars

Other Positive Health Effects - Five Stars

Method - Vitamin E tocotrienols are almost always made from one of three sources: rice, palm oil, or annato. The best source is palm oil tocotrienols, because they have the best mix of individual elements (alpha, beta, gamma, and delta). The palm oil tocotrienols are also the same types that were shown to re-grow hair in the research. I take NSI brand, but a few others make almost the same product. Many are called Tocomin Suprabio, because this is the source that they get it from. Take around 100mg of total tocotrienols per day, which is usually two pills worth.

Laser Treatment

Scientific Evidence - Four Stars

Web Testimonials - Three Stars

Author's Experience - N/A

Expense - Three Stars (large one time expense)

Other Positive Health Effects - Two Stars

Method - Purchase a Hair Laser Comb, or similar device. Ratings for individual machines are available at amazon.com. Search for the Laser Comb, and then see similar products. Follow directions on the package. You can also use the YellowPages or an internet search to find a hair laser treatment center near you.

Toppik

Scientific Evidence - N/A but the product clearly works

Web Testimonials - Five Stars

Author's Experience - N/A

Expense - Two Stars

Other Positive Health Effects - One Stars

Method - Buy Toppik powder and apply using the instructions on the package. This product fuses to your existing hair and appears to be your own hair, but fuller and thicker, and covering up minor to moderate (but not large) bald spots. Toppik looks great, and is worth it if nothing else works, or if you need temporary help while trying several of the above solutions. It washes out in the shower.

7. CONCLUDING

You can see from the rating guide that there are no options that got a full five stars for scientific evidence. Keep in mind this is in regards to current scientific evidence, because if those that had one positive trial done on humans get another one done, then it will move into the five star evidence range.

You can also see that none of the therapies have a five star rating from my own personal experience. I think that this goes to show the nature of natural therapies. Instead of being thought of as "silver bullet" therapies, natural therapies in most cases are simply what the body wanted to have in the first place.

In other words, losing hair might be the body's warning that it didn't have the correct fatty acids as the resources for it to run properly. Replacing just fish oil won't cut it - you will have made significant progress only when you replace all of the proper fatty acids.

Or, losing hair might be the symptom of not eating whole grains which naturally contain phytates, or IP6. The body expects these phytates to be in the diet so that it can clear out excess calcium that is choking off the hair and leading to other health issues. Replacing IP6 restores the body to how it should have been in the first place.

Or hair loss could be due to the fact that minerals that the body was supposed to be getting, like silica or iodine, simply weren't available in the diet. Replacing them through optimal supplementation just brings the body back into a state of sufficiency, or how it wanted to be in the first place.

You can see why, through all of these natural therapies, not only is your hair repaired, but your whole body is able to work better using a complete set of nutrients that it needs. Contrast that with drug therapy that has the underlying mission to simply mask the problem, altering bodily activities while still running at a deficit of nutrients. In a long-term situation, you can see why this is unhealthy, and why following the rules of this book may be the key to great health for you, both for your hair and otherwise.

ENDNOTES

[1] Jordan, V.E. (1976). Protein status of the elderly as measured by dietary intake, hair tissue, and serum albumin. American Journal of Clinical Nutrition, 29(5), 522-8. Available http://www.ncbi.nlm.nih.gov/pubmed/1266793

[2] Biolo, G. & Guadagni, M. (2009) Effects of inflammation and/or inactivity on the need for dietary protein. Current Opinion in Clinical Nutrition and Metabolic Care, 12(6), 617-22. Available http://www.ncbi.nlm.nih.gov/pubmed/19741515

[3] Liang, T., & Liao, S. (1992). Inhibition of steroid 5 alpha-reductase by specific aliphatic unsaturated fatty acids. The Biochemical Journal, (Pt 2), 557-62. Available http://www.ncbi.nlm.nih.gov/pubmed/1637346

[4] Kondo, R., Shimizu, K., & Liu, J. (2009). Anti-androgenic activity of fatty acids. Chemistry and Biodiversity Journal, 6(4), 503-12. Available http://www.ncbi.nlm.nih.gov/pubmed/19353546

[5] Cousse, H., Martin, P.M., & Raynaud, J.P. (2002). Inhibition of type 1 and type 2 5alpha-reductase activity by free fatty acids, active ingredients of Permixon. Journal of Steroid Biochemistry and Molecular Biology, 82(2-3), 233-9. Available http://www.ncbi.nlm.nih.gov/pubmed/12477490

[6] Ehrlich, S. (2011). Omega-6 fatty acids. University of Maryland Medical Center. Available http://www.umm.edu/altmed/articles/omega-6-000317.htm

[7] Chang, J. (2008). Estrogen dominance, women's problems, amenorrhea, and menopause. Sensible Health. Available http://www.sensiblehealth.com/Journey-04.xhtml

[8] Assuncao, M.L., Ferreira, H.S., et al. (2009). Effects of dietary coconut oil on the biochemical and anthropometric profiles of women presenting abdominal obesity. Lipids Journal, 44(7), 593-601. Available http://www.ncbi.nlm.nih.gov/pubmed/19437058

[9] Rele, A.S., & Mohile, R.B. (2003). Effect of mineral oil, sunflower oil, and coconut oil on prevention of hair damage. Journal of Cosmetic Science, 54(2), 175-92. Available http://www.ncbi.nlm.nih.gov/pubmed/12715094

[10] Gallego-Lago, J.L., Rico, H., et al. (2000). Effect of silicon supplement on osteopenia induced by ovariectomy in rats. Calcified Tissue International Journal, 66(1), 53-5. Available http://www.ncbi.nlm.nih.gov/pubmed/10602845

[11] Kossmann, K., Wickett, R.R., et al. (2007). Effect of oral intake of choline-stabilized orthosilicic acid on hair tensile strength and morphology in women with fine hair.

Archives of Dermatological Research, 299(10), 499-505.
Available
http://www.ncbi.nlm.nih.gov/pubmed/17960402

[12] Rushton, D.H. (2003). Decreased serum ferritin is
associated with alopecia in women. Journal of
Investigative Dermatology, 121(5), 985-8. Available
http://www.ncbi.nlm.nih.gov/pubmed/14708596

[13] Eckman, A., & Zieve, D. (2010). Hypothyroidism.
PubMed Health. Available
http://www.ncbi.nlm.nih.gov/pubmedhealth/PMH00013
93/

[14] Irwig, M.S., & Kolukula, S. (2011). Persistent sexual side
effects of finasteride for male pattern hair loss. The
Journal of Sexual Medicine, 8(6), 1747-53. Available
http://www.ncbi.nlm.nih.gov/pubmed/21418145

[15] Di Silverio, F., Monti, S., et al. (1998). Effects of long-
term treatment with Serenoa repens (Permixon) on the
concentrations and regional distribution of androgens
and epidermal growth factor in benign prostatic
hyperplasia. The Prostate Journal, 37(2), 77-83. Available
http://www.ncbi.nlm.nih.gov/pubmed/9759701

[16] Zhou, J., Lunyin, Y., et al. (2003). Soy Phytochemicals
and Tea Bioactive Components Synergistically Inhibit
Androgen-Sensitive Human Prostate Tumors in Mice.
Journal of Nutrition, 133(2), 516-521. Available
http://www.ncbi.nlm.nih.gov/pmc/articles/PMC2683253

[17] Capodice, J., Stone, B., & Katz, A. (2009). Evaluation of an At-Home-Use Prostate Massage Device for Men with Lower Urinary Tract Symptoms. The Open Urology & Nephrology Journal, 2, 20-23. Available http://www.highisland.com/images/20TOUNJ.pdf

[18] Hoelzel, F. (1942). Baldness and Calcification of the "Ivory Dome." Journal of the American Medical Association, 119(12), 968. Available http://jama.ama-assn.org/content/119/12/968.3.short

[19] Vucenik, I., and Shamsuddin, A.M. (2003). Cancer Inhibition by Inositol Hexaphosphate (IP6) and Inositol: From Laboratory to Clinic. The Journal of Nutrition, 133(11), 37785-37845. Available http://jn.nutrition.org/content/133/11/3778S.full

[20] Grases, F., & Costa-Bauza, A. (1999). Phytate (IP6) is a powerful agent for preventing calcifications in biological flduis: usefulness in renal Lithia sis treatment. Anticancer Research Journal, 19(5A), 3717-22. Available http://www.ncbi.nlm.nih.gov/pubmed/10625946

[21] Grases, F. Prieto, R.M., et al. (2008). Role of phytate and osteopontin in the mechanism of soft tissue calcification. Journal of Nephrology, 21(5), 768-75. Available http://www.ncbi.nlm.nih.gov/pubmed/18949733

[22] Vermeer, C., & Geleijnse, J.M. (2004). Dietary intake of menaquinone is associated with a reduced risk of

97

coronary heart disease. The Journal of Nutrition, 134(11), 3100-5. Available http://www.ncbi.nlm.nih.gov/pubmed/15514282

[23] Ezaki, J., Koitaya, N., et al. (2009). Effect of low dose vitamin K2 (MK-4) supplementation on bio-indices in post-menopausal Japanese women. Journal of Nutritional Science and Vitaminology, 55(1), 15-21. Available http://www.ncbi.nlm.nih.gov/pubmed/19352059

[24] Vorvick, L.J., Berman, K., & Zieve, D. (2010). Alopecia Areata. Pubmed Health. Available http://www.ncbi.nlm.nih.gov/pubmedhealth/pmh000242 1/

[25] Hay, I.C., Jamieson, M., & Ormerod, A.D. (1998). Randomized Trial of Aromatherapy: Successful Treatment for Alopecia Areata. Archives of Dermatology, 134(11), 1349-1352. Available http://archderm.ama-assn.org/cgi/content/full/134/11/1349

[26] Henley, D., Lipson, N., et al. (2007). Prepubertal Gynecomastia Linked to Lavender and Tea Tree Oils. New England Journal of Medicine, 356, 479-485. Available http://www.nejm.org/doi/full/10.1056/NEJMoa064725

[27] Kamiya, T., Takahashi, T., & Yokoo, Y. (1998). Proanthocyanidins from grape seeds promote proliferation of mouse hair follicle cells in vitro and convert hair cycle in vivo. Acta Dermato-Venereologica,

78(6), 428-32. Available
http://www.ncbi.nlm.nih.gov/pubmed/9833041

[28] Kamiya, T., Takahashi, T., et al. (1999). Procyanidin oligomers selectively and intensively promote proliferation of mouse hair epithelial cells in vitro and activate hair follicle growth in vivo. The Journal of Investigative Dermatology, 112(3), 310-6. Available http://www.ncbi.nlm.nih.gov/pubmed/10084307

[29] Ehrlich, S. (2011). Grape Seed. University of Maryland Medical Center. Available http://www.umm.edu/altmed/articles/grape-seed-000254.htm

[30] Nakamura, Y., Tsuji, S., & Tonogai, Y. (2003). Analysis of Proanthocyanidins in Grape Seed Extracts, Health Foods and Grape Seed Oils. Journal of Health Science, 49(1), 45-54. Available http://jhs.pharm.or.jp/data/49(1)/49_45.pdf

[31] Matsuda, H., Yamazaki, M., et al. (2003). Promotion of hair growth by ginseng radix on cultured mouse vibrissal hair follicles. Phytotherapy Research Journal, 17(7), 797-800. Available http://www.ncbi.nlm.nih.gov/pubmed/12916080

[32] Park, S., Shin, W.S., & Ho, J. (2011). Fructus panax ginseng extract promotes hair regeneration in C57BL/6 mice. Journal of Ethnopharmacology, Epub. Available http://www.ncbi.nlm.nih.gov/pubmed/21959181

[33] Li, F., Tan, W., et al. (2010). Tocotrienol enriched palm oil prevents atherosclerosis though modulating the activities of peroxisome proliferators-activated receptors. Atherosclerosis Journal, 211(1), 278-82. Available http://www.ncbi.nlm.nih.gov/pubmed/20138624

[34] Fang, F., Kang, Z., & Wong, C. Vitamin E tocotrienols improve insulin sensitivity through activating peroxisome proliferator-activated receptors. Molecular Nutrition and Food Research Journal, 54(3), 345-52. Available http://www.ncbi.nlm.nih.gov/pubmed/19866471

[35] Sylvester, P.W., Wali, V.B., et al. (2011). Tocotrienol combination therapy results in synergistic anticancer response. Frontiers in Bioscience: A Journal and Virtual Library, 17, 3183-95. Available http://www.ncbi.nlm.nih.gov/pubmed/21622228

[36] Ai Beoy, L., Jia Woei, W., & Kah Hay. (2010). Effects on Tocotrienol Supplementation on Hair Growth in Human Volunteers. Tropical Life Sciences Research, 21(2), 95-103. Available http://www.tlsr.usm.my/earlyviewDetail_files/ARTICLES/TLSR%2021-2-8-Lim.pdf

[37] Charles, G., Leavitt, M., et al. (2009). HairMax LaserComb laser phototherapy device in the treatment of male androgenetic alopecia: A randomized, double-blind, sham device-controlled, multicoated trial. Clinical Drug Investigation Journal, 29(5), 283-92. Available http://www.ncbi.nlm.nih.gov/pubmed/19366270

For More Natural Health Information from David Rodgers, including the free report "Diet Soda Makes You Fatter Than Regular and 10 More Shocking Health Truths," visit www.nutrientbalance.com

About the Author

David Rodgers received his Masters of Science in Human Nutrition from the University of Bridgeport, one of the nation's foremost regionally accredited universities focused on natural health.

Prior to and concurrent with his degree program, David spent a large portion of ten years researching, analyzing, and synthesizing texts and research journals dealing with the effects that nutrition, vitamins, minerals, amino acids, fatty acids, probiotics, phytochemicals, herbs, exercise, and lifestyle measures have on people's health. Upon finding all of the above measures have profound effects on the body and specifically chronic disease, he decided to formalize his education and start a clinic known as the Nutrient Balance Center.

In addition to hair loss, David specializes in helping people with Chronic Lyme Disease, chronic fatigue syndrome, fibromyalgia, lupus, and multiple sclerosis using all natural dietary, supplemental, and lifestyle measures.

More information is available at www.nutrientbalance.com.